Consumer's Guide to Fruits and Vegetables

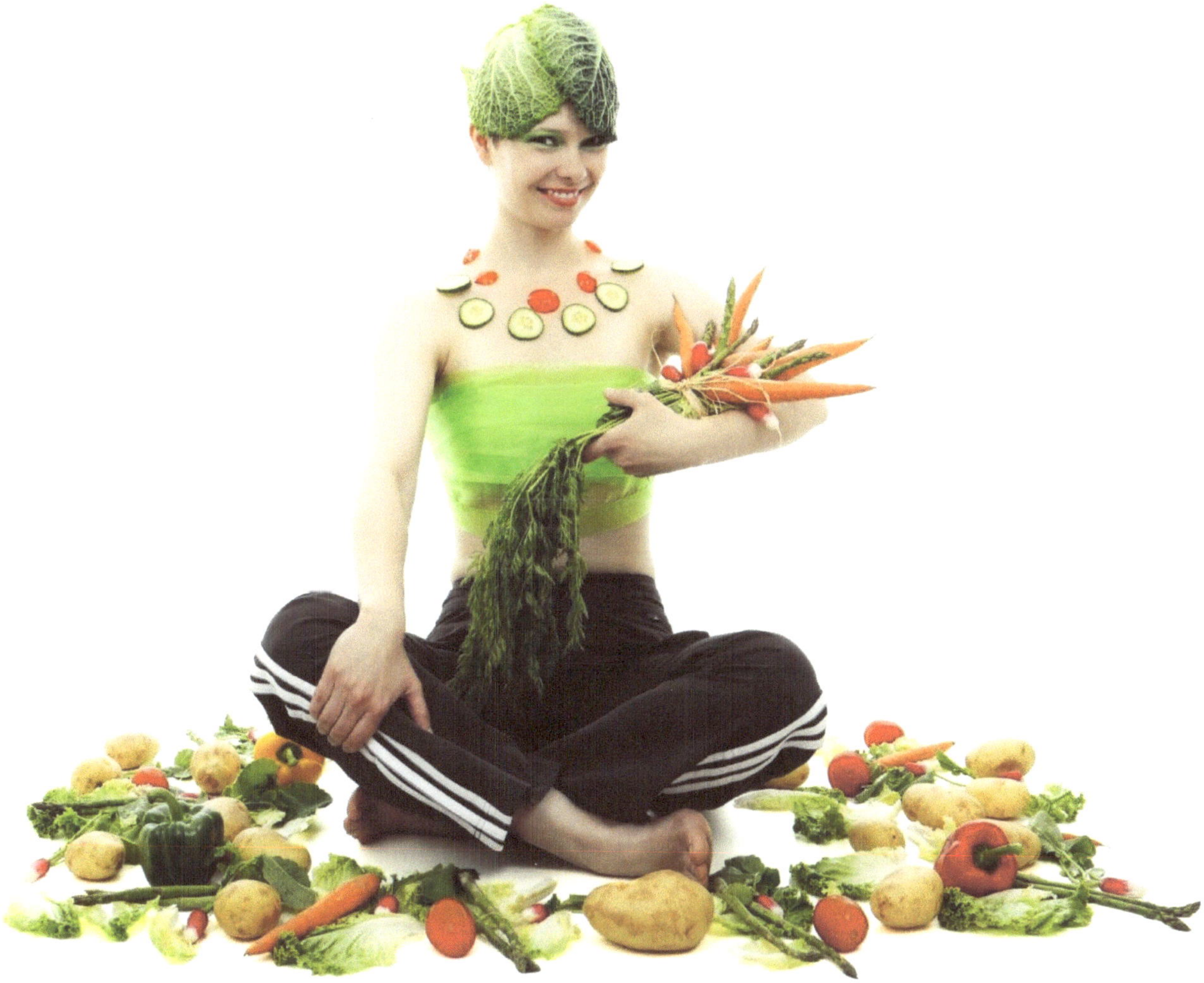

By Mae Gardner

ISBN: 1511515759
ISBN 13: 9781511515757

Introduction

This book was prepared to guide consumers with the healthy foods to maintain better health. A good diet along with proper nutrients will help the immune system to heal naturally. Essential nutrients are needed daily to allow the body to function mentally and physically.

The images on each page describe the fruits and vegetables. They also explain some vitamins and minerals contained in the foods and their functions in the body.

The book has been created in large print for convenience to senior citizens as well as individuals with eye problems.

Asparagus ………………………………………. Nectarine

Broccoli……………………………………….. Onion

Carrot……………………………………… Potato

Dandelion……………………………………….. Quince

Egg Plant……………………………………… Radish

Fennel…………………………………………… Squash

Garlic………………………………………. Tomato

Habanero Pepper…………………………….… Ugli

Indian Corn……………………………………… Voavanga

Jack Bean…………………………………….... Watermelon

Kale…………………………………………..... Xigua

Lettuce………………………………………… Yams

Mushroom…………………………………….... Zucchini

Vital Nutrients for a Healthy Adult Diet

Protein
The average adult female needs 46 grams of protein daily, while the average adult male requires 56 grams. An individual can obtain his or her recommended dietary allowance (RDA) of vitamins by eating foods listed below:

Almonds	Hemp Seeds
Berries	Kale
Brussel Sprouts	Oats
Flax Seeds or Oil	Spinach
Green leafy Vegetables	Sunflower Seed

Calcium
Helps to build strong bones when taken with vitamin D and a bone building mineral like magnesium.   It is found in:

Broccoli	Figs
Collards	Kale

Vitamin D can be obtained by spending time in the sun daily or by taking a vitamin D supplement.
Magnesium is a bone building mineral which also supports the skin and heart.
The best sources are:

Almonds	Cucumber
Apples	Figs
Bananas	Onion
Beets	Oranges
Celery	Spinach

Our bodies also require Iron to move oxygen through the blood and helps in building red blood cells. The best sources are:

Broccoli	Romaine Lettuce
Kale	Salads
Pumpkin Seeds	Sunflower Seeds

An essential Fatty Acid is Omega 3 it reduces inflammation, pain, reduces the risk of heart disease, strokes and improves brain function.

Sources for Omega 3 are:

Broccoli	Green Leafy Vegetables
Flax Seeds	Walnuts

Consumer's Guide to Fruits & Vegetables, A to Z

Asparagus

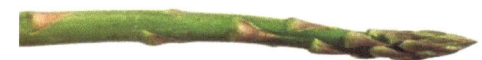

One serving of asparagus has only 20 calories, no fat or cholesterol, 5 mg.   of sodium, 400 mg. of potassium, 5 grams of fiber, 60% of the USRDA   of folacin, which is necessary for the formation of blood cells, growth,   and prevention of liver disease.

Asparagus was first cultivated about 2500 years ago in Greece. In their conquests, the Romans spread it to the Gauls, Germans, Britons, and from there the rest of the world.

Broccoli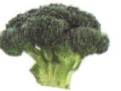

Broccoli gives us nutrition and helps our body fight diseases. This vegetable is high in vitamin C and dietary fiber. A single serving of broccoli provides 30 mg of vitamin C.

Broccoli also contains multiple nutrients with potent anti-cancer properties.

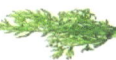

Carrot

Carrots provide us with nutrients for healthy hair, eyes, skin, bones and mucous membranes.

The carrot gets its bright orange color from beta-carotene. Alpha and beta carotenes are partly metabolized into vitamin A in humans. Good for Bugs Bunny, good for kids.

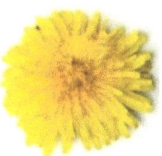

Dandelions

Dandelions are wild plants grown in rural areas and farm locations. They supply vitamin A, C, and K. In the Eurasian countries they are cultivated for human consumption. The flower petals of dandelions are used to make dandelion wine and are one of the ingredients of root beer.

Some people consider dandelion a weed; some consider it a flower.

Egg Plants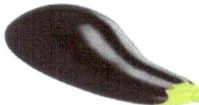

Egg plants are used mostly for vegetarian and ethnic dishes. They are low in calories unless cooked in fat.

Which came first, the chicken or the eggplant?

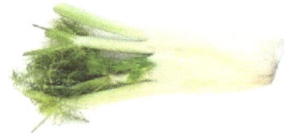

Fennels

Fennels contain vitamins A and C, potassium, calcium, iron and fiber. The bulb, foliage and seeds are widely used in many of the culinary traditions of the world. For cooking, the bulb is a crisp vegetable that can be sautéed, stewed, braised, or eaten raw.

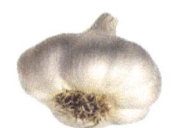

Garlic

Garlic is widely used around the world for its pungent flavor as a seasoning or condiment. Garlic bulbs are normally divided into numerous fleshy sections called cloves. These cloves are consumed (raw or cooked) or for medicinal purposes. Garlic can be applied to different kinds of bread to create a variety of classic dishes such as garlic bread, garlic toast, etc.

One of the drawbacks to eating garlic, of course, is that it causes "bad" breath (halitosis). But in 1924 it was found to prevent scurvy because of its high vitamin C content.

Habanero Peppers

Habanero peppers are both hot and healthy. They are high in minerals and vitamins C and A. Capsaicin, the active "hot" chemical in habaneros, kills unwanted bacteria and intestinal parasites.

How hot is a habanero? A jalapeno pepper has an SHU (Scoville hot unit) of 5,000 and a habanero has an SHU of 200,000. That's hot.

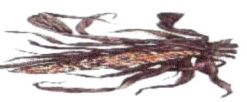

Indian corn

Indian corn (flint corn) is one of three types of corn that was cultivated by Native Americans, both in New England and across the northern tier, including tribes such as the Pawnee on the Great Plains. Indian corn is the type of corn preferred for making hominy, and it is sometimes called "ornamental" corn because of its use in Thanksgiving decorations in the United States.

Because Indian corn has a very low water content it is more resistant to freezing than other vegetables. It was the only Vermont crop to survive New England's infamous "Year without a summer" of 1816.

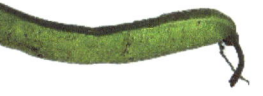

Jack Beans

Jack bean, canavalia ensiformis, is a legume which is used for animal fodder and human nutrition. In the United States, it is cultivated mainly in the southern states for animal fodder.

Kale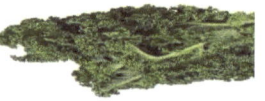

Kale is a vegetable similar to cabbage, with green or purple leaves, in which the central leaves do not form a head. Kale is very high in beta carotene, vitamin K, C, and E, and is rich in calcium.

Kale freezes well and actually tastes sweeter and more flavorful after being exposed to frost.

Lettuce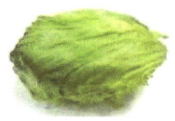

Lettuce contains vitamin A, C, K, Calcium, Iron, and Potassium, with a higher concentration of vitamins found in darker green lettuce. Lettuce is most often used in salads, although it is also used in soups, sandwiches, and wraps.

Despite its beneficial properties, lettuce, when contaminated is often a source of bacterial, viral, and parasitic outbreaks in humans, including E. coli, and salmonella.

Mushrooms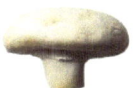

Edible mushrooms are the fleshy and edible fruit bodies of several species of fungi.
Before assuming that any wild mushroom is edible it should be identified, because many species are very toxic to humans and can be very poisonous. As a rule all wild mushrooms should be cooked thoroughly before eating.

Nectarine

A nectarine is rich in fiber, vitamin A, vitamin C, vitamin E, and potassium.

A nectarine has smooth skin and is sometimes called a "shaved peach" because of its lack of fuzz or short hairs. It is sometimes erroneously believed to be a cross between a peach and a plum. But though fuzzy peaches and nectarines are regarded commercially as different fruits, the nectarine is just a different species of peach.

Onion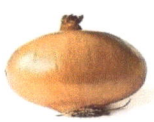

dietary fiber. They also contain chemical compounds such as phenolics and flavonoids that have potential anti-inflammatory, anti-cholesterol, anticancer and antioxidant properties.

In the middle Ages onions were such an important food that people would pay their rent with onions, and even give them as gifts. According to diaries kept by early colonists in America, bulb onions were one of the first things planted by the Pilgrim Fathers when they cleared the land for cropping in 1648.

Potato

A medium sized potato with skin provides 27 mg of vitamin C (45 % of the daily value), and 620 mg of potassium (18 % of DV). The potato is best known for its carbohydrate content (about 26 grams in a medium potato).

Potatoes are the world's fourth-largest food crop, following rice, wheat, and maize (corn). Humans can survive healthily on a diet of potatoes supplemented only with milk or butter which contain the two vitamins not provided by potatoes: vitamin A and D.

Quince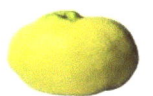

Quince is high in carbohydrates, vitamin C (18% DV), calcium, potassium, and dietary fiber. The U.S. gets most of its quince from Argentina.

High in pectin, quince fruit is used to make jam and jelly. Originally, marmalade was made from quince fruit.

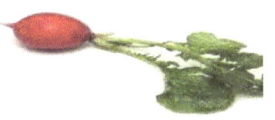

Radish

Radishes are a good source of vitamin B6 and vitamin C, and are rich in ascorbic acid, folic acid, potassium and calcium. There are many varieties of radishes, but the most common radish seen in supermarkets in North America is the Cherry Belle, a bright red-skinned round variety.

The radish is a root plant; therefore insects can attack the leaves all day long with little effect on the edible root, which makes it a good companion plant for more vulnerable vegetables—sort of like a decoy.

Squash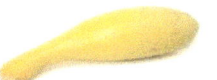

Squash is a source of many vitamins and minerals, with a high percentage of vitamin C (20%), vitamin B6 (17%) and riboflavin (12%).

Squash was one of the "Three Sisters" planted by Native Americans. These were the three main native crop plants: maize (corn), beans, and squash. They were usually planted together, with the corn stalk serving as support for the climbing beans, and shade for the squash.

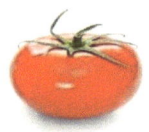

Tomato

The tomato contains a powerful antioxidant, lycopene, and provides a high percentage of vitamin C, A, B6, and A, as well as many beneficial minerals such as potassium and manganese.

While the tomato is a fruit, it is considered a vegetable for culinary purposes. The Tariff Act of 1883 required a tax to be paid on imported vegetables but not fruit, so the U.S. Supreme Court ruled that the tomato should be classified under customs regulation as a vegetable instead of a fruit. Tricky stuff, huh? Botanically a tomato *is* a fruit because it is a seed-bearing structure growing from the flowering part of a plant.

Ugli

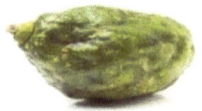

A single serving of Ugli fruit contains an amazing 70% of the recommended daily value of vitamin C to your diet.

UGLI is a trademark of Cold Hall Citrus Limited and under which it sells its Jamaican tangelo, a citrus fruit that is a cross between a grapefruit, an orange, and a tangerine. It was discovered growing wild in Jamaica by the people who, after an importer said, "…send me some more of that *ugly* fruit," changed its name to UGLI and developed it commercially.

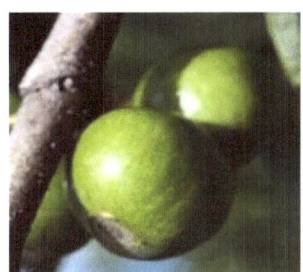

Voavanga

Little is known in the United States about the nutritional value of the Voavanga (Spanish tamarind). It is said to be native to Mexico.

The Voavanga is a green round fruit with white dots. It turns brown when ripe.

Watermelon

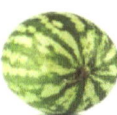

A watermelon contains about 6% sugar and 91% water by weight, and like many other fruits it is a source of vitamin C (10% of daily requirements).

A lot of bees are required to pollinate a watermelon patch. The US Department of Agriculture recommends that for commercial planting one beehive per acre be provided for pollination of watermelons, and three beehives per acre for seedless watermelons because seedless varieties have sterile pollen.

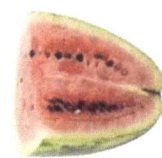

Xigua

Xigua is an African name for watermelon, the same watermelon pictured on the previous page, according to many sources. However, one source of information describes the xigua as an African melon like the watermelon except smaller and shorter in length. One fact they all agree on is that the watermelon, by whatever name, originated in Africa. Another fact we all can agree on is that the xigua starts with the letter X, thus fulfilling the alphabetical need of this book.

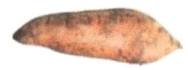

Yams

Yams (sweet potatoes) are rich in vitamins A, C, and B6, beta-carotene, and potassium. In 1992 the nutritional value of sweet potatoes was compared to other vegetables. Considering fiber content, complex carbohydrates, protein, vitamins A and C, iron and calcium, the sweet potato was the highest in nutritional value with a score of 184, more than a hundred points higher than the next on the list, the common potato.

Yams are native to Africa, where 95% of them are grown. They are not sweet potatoes. However, the "soft" varieties of sweet potatoes are often called yams in the United States. So if you are eating a yam in the U.S. you are probably eating a sweet potato.

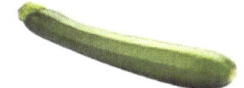

Zucchini

 The zucchini squash is low in calories. It contains significant amounts of folate, potassium, and vitamin A.

 The zucchini squash is a fruit; however it is treated as a vegetable for culinary purposes. While easy to grow, zucchini, like all squash, requires plentiful bees for pollination.

Recipes

Spinach Salad
Serve 4

$\frac{1}{2}$ lb. Spinach
3 slices bread (diced in $\frac{1}{2}$ inch cubes
$\frac{1}{2}$ Cup Salad oil

Brown bread in skillet or toast
Put into a bowl and sprinkle with garlic and $\frac{1}{4}$ cup parmesan cheese, let cool. Add $\frac{1}{2}$ cup French Salad dressing and Spinach, (wilt)

Asparagus Casserole
Serve 6

1 can or fresh Asparagus
1 can Mushroom Soup
$\frac{1}{2}$ lbs. grated Cheese
4 hardboiled eggs (chopped)
Cracker crumbs

Arrange layers of Asparagus, Cheese, eggs, and soup in oiled casserole Dish, top with cracker crumbs

Bake at 350 degrees temperature for 20 minutes

Healthy Mary
Serve 2

3 Cups chopped tomatoes
1 Cup Water
½ Cup chopped red bell pepper
1 ½ tablespoon fresh grated horseradish root
1 Jalapeno Pepper (seeded)
1 small clove garlic
1 teaspoon tamarind paste
½ teaspoon celery (chopped)
¼ teaspoon sea salt

Cayenne and fresh ground pepper to taste
Put ingredients into blender and blend until smooth and serve
Celery stalk and lime wedge for garnish
To make a green Mary add spinach.

Watermelon-Fennel-Mint Chiller

4 Cups Watermelon (cubed)
1 Cup fennel, white bulb only (chopped)
½ Cup fresh mints (loosely packed)

Place in blender and process until frothy. Serve

Note: Watermelon contains more lycopene than tomatoes, and are believed to be an excellent source of vitamin C and beta carotene which is believed to improve kidney function.

Chicken Pies
Serve 6

3 ounces cream cheese
1 teaspoon chopped chives
½ Cup butter (melt)
1 Cup all-purpose flour
½ teaspoon salt

Place cream cheese, chives and butter in mixing bowl. Blend until creamy Add flour and salt, blend well. Form into a ball, cover and chill.

HISTORY

"WILD FRUITS OF THE COUNTRYSIDE"

WILD FRUITS OF THE COUNTRYSIDE

1. Cloudberry.   2. Crab Apple.   3. Sweetbriar Fruit.   4. Privet Fruit.   5. Strawberry-tree Fruit (E.).
6. Spurge Laurel (E.).   7. Acorns.   8. Common Barberry.   9. Whortleberry.   10. Butcher's Broom (E.).
Plants marked (E.) are European and are not generally found in America.

4021

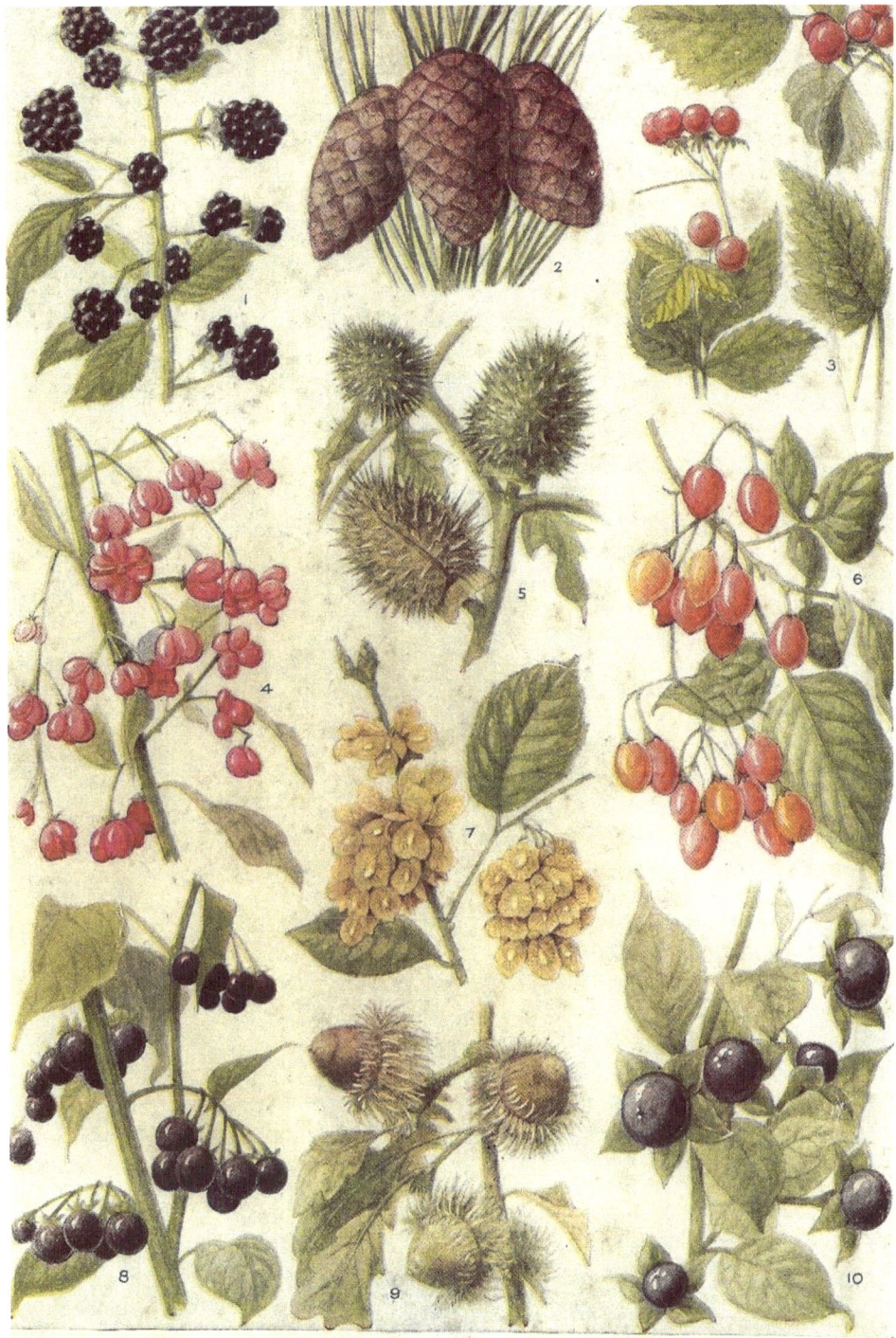

1. Blackberry.   2. Scotch Pine.   3. Roebuck-berry, or Stone Bramble (E.).   4. Common Spindle Tree.
5. Thorn Apple.   6. Bitter-sweet.   7. Common English Elm.   8. Black Solanum, or Nightshade.
9. Turkey, or Moss-cupped Oak (E.).   10. Deadly Nightshade, or Dwale (E.).

4028

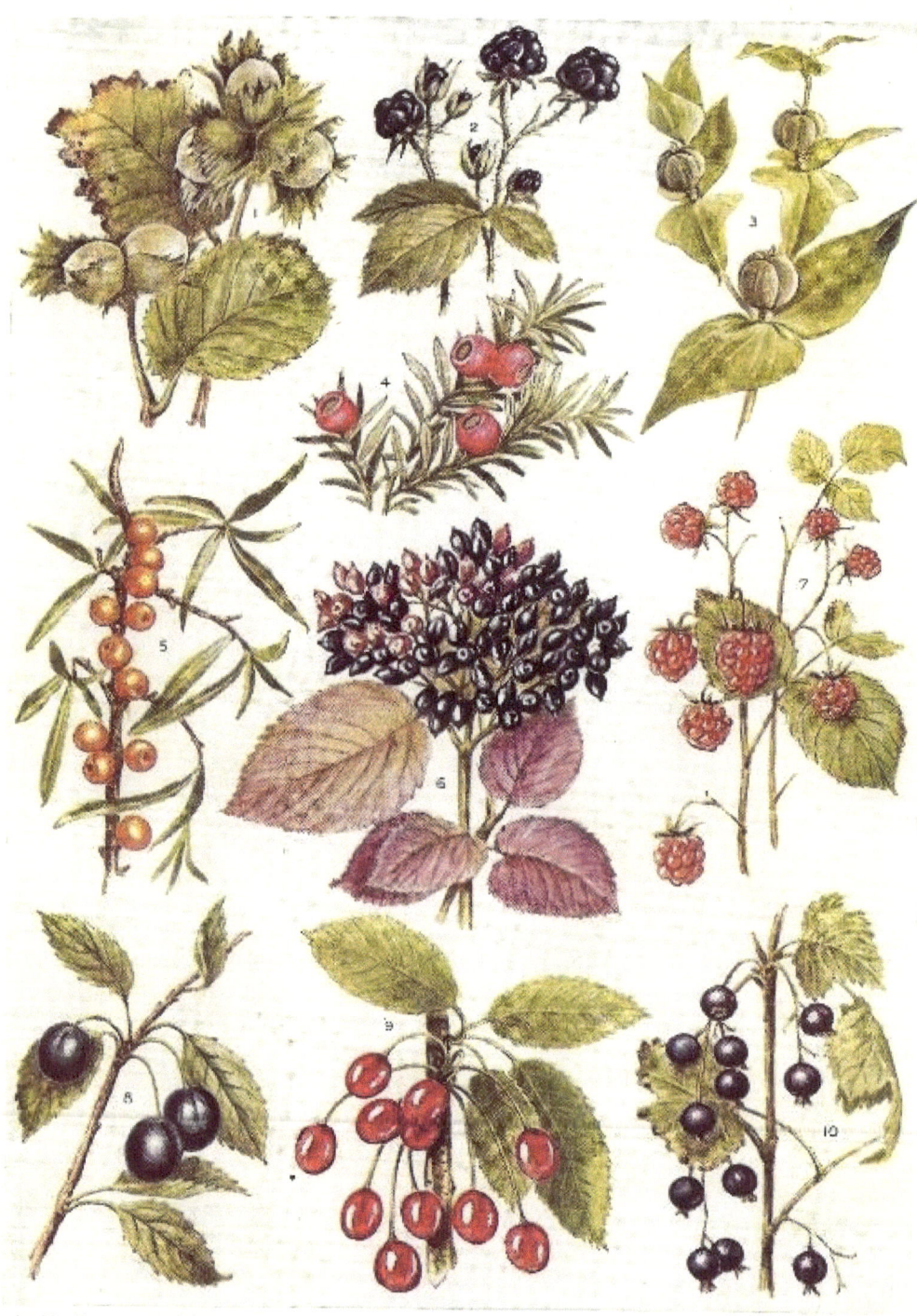

1. Hazel. 2. Dewberry. 3. Caper Spurge. 4. Yew (E.). 5. Sea Buckthorn. 6. Wayfaring Tree (E.). 7. Red Raspberry. 8. Bullace (E.). 9. Wild Red Cherry. 10. Wild Black Currant.

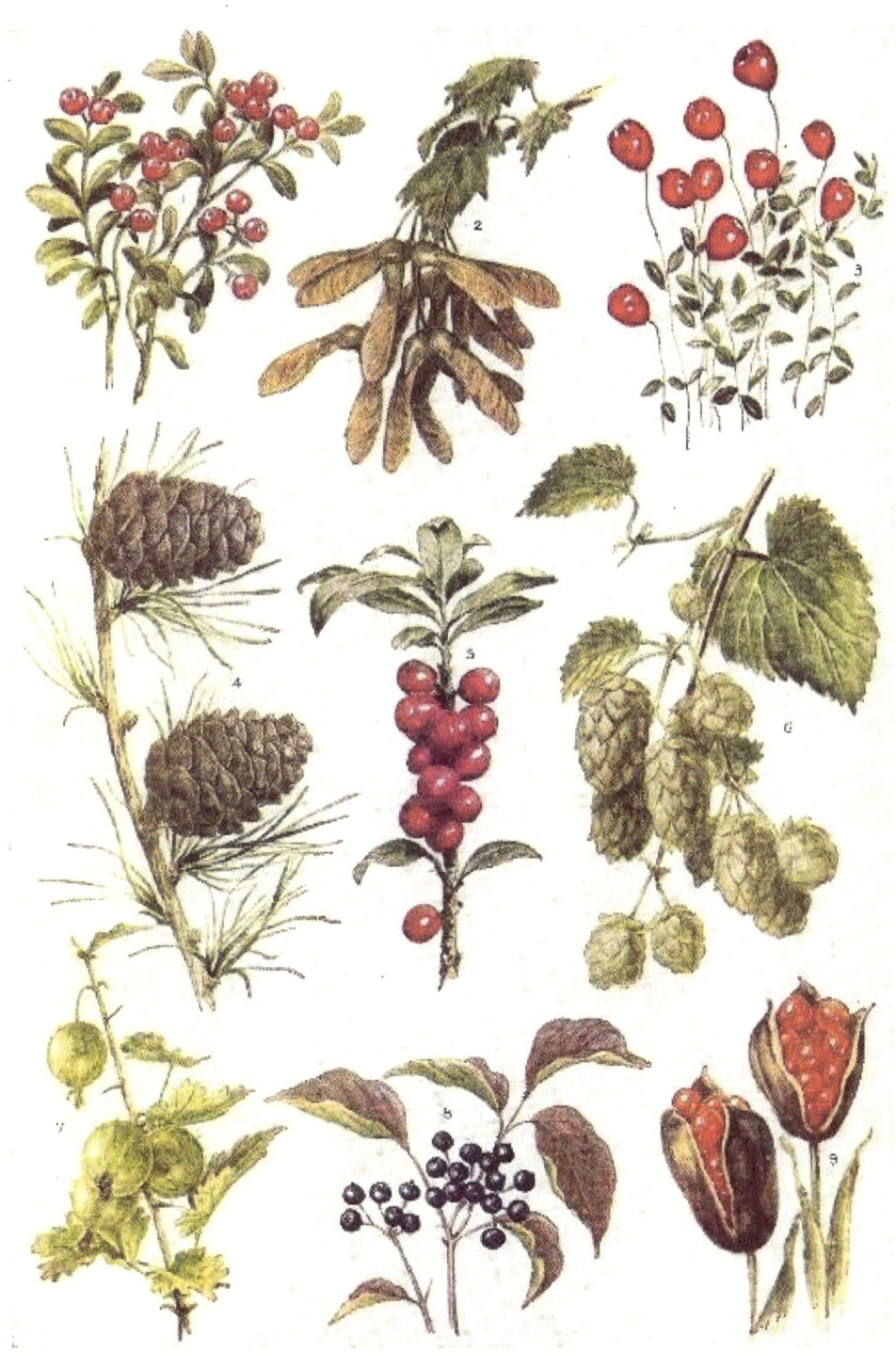

1. Common Bearberry. 2. Maple. 3. Cranberry. 4. Larch. 5. Mezereon (E.). 6. Hops. 7. Gooseberry. 8. Dogwood. 9. Fetid Iris (E.).

4022

Our acknowledgement of the wealth of information we gathered from Wikipedia online encyclopedia and English Dictionary Second Edition. Bell, Stacey 2010. Nutritional Healing – Fifth Edition. New York: (Penguin Group (USA)

And, of course, many thanks to Google.